HOLISTIC APPROACH TO LYME DISEASE

A Comprehensive Integrative Approach to
Diagnosing and Treating Tick-Borne Illness

I0454209

Isabella White

Disclaimer: The information in this book is based on the author's research, opinions, and experiences. It is not intended to replace professional medical advice or treatment. The reader should regularly consult a physician for any health issues and always seek the advice of a physician before modifying diet, supplement, or exercise regimens. The author and publisher shall have neither liability nor responsibility to any person or entity concerning any loss or damage related to the information contained in this book. The information provided is general and may not apply to every individual. Any reliance on the information contained herein is solely at the reader's risk.

Table of Contents

Introduction

Lyme disease has only been recognized in modern medicine for about 50 years, but its origins extend further. Cases resembling what we now call Lyme have been documented as far back as the late 19th century in Europe. However, it was not until the 1970s, when a cluster of pediatric arthritis cases were noted in Lyme, Connecticut, that medical experts began investigating what we recognize today as Lyme disease.

The culprit behind Lyme is the aptly named bacteria Borrelia burgdorferi, which is transmitted to humans through tick bites. Blacklegged ticks infected with B. burgdorferi initially transmit the pathogen while in their nymph stage—tiny, juvenile ticks roughly the size of a poppy seed. Due to their diminutive size, nymphal ticks often go unnoticed when latching on for a blood meal, allowing ample time to transmit the bacteria. Once inside the human body, B. burgdorferi migrates through tissue and blood to cause various symptoms.

While antibiotics are often effective for treatment in the early stages, Lyme has a habit of burrowing deep into tissues. This can allow it to persist despite antibiotic therapy and continue triggering symptoms for months or years afterward. With cases on the rise and traditional medicine still catching up, this complex, often misdiagnosed disease demands a holistic, patient-focused approach like the one outlined in this book.

This book aims to provide Lyme disease patients and practitioners with a roadmap to genuinely and holistically diagnosing and treating this complex illness. Conventional medicine often falls short of effectively and compassionately caring for Lyme patients. Labels like "post-treatment Lyme disease syndrome" minimize patient experiences and leave many without solutions for their ongoing symptoms.

This book aims to rectify that deficiency by highlighting integrative diagnostic methods beyond simple blood testing and evidence-based complementary treatments to pair with antibiotics or employ when antibiotics fail. The latest insights from top Lyme-literate meds will be distilled along with nutritional and lifestyle measures patients can enact to empower themselves.

It is time for an integrated, patient-centered approach to become the standard for understanding and managing tick-borne illnesses. This book will focus on giving patients and practitioners the tools to make that happen. Most importantly, it is intended to offer hope grounded in science and compassion to those Lyme sufferers who have wandered the medical wilderness for far too long without answers. This book illuminates the path home.

Chapter 1

Understanding Lyme Disease

The Science Behind Lyme Disease

Lyme disease progresses in three stages: early localized infection, early disseminated infection, and potentially late dissemination involving the nervous system and joints. Understanding this progression helps inform diagnostics and treatment.

In early localized Lyme, the Borrelia burgdorferi (Bb) bacteria transmitted from an infected tick bite first migrate through the skin before entering the bloodstream. Flu-like symptoms often emerge as the immune system responds to the foreign invader. If untreated, Bb will disseminate through the blood and lymph nodes, potentially causing arrhythmias or nerve pain.

Weeks later, late-disseminated Lyme can develop as bacteria hide from immune cells, allowing them to damage tissues and trigger inflammatory responses, explaining the joint pain and cognitive dysfunction many experience. Bb is known to drill into cartilage and other collagenous tissues. It may also traverse the blood-brain barrier and invade the central nervous system.

While the exact mechanisms of persistent symptomology are still being unraveled, researchers suspect Bb can alter gene transcription once inside human cells and shift immune functioning out of homeostasis. By understanding Lyme's pathogenesis within the body, we can better direct testing and tailor treatment for patients suffering acute infections or wrestling with lingering effects.

Historical Perspective

While Lyme disease, as we define it today, has only been studied for around 50 years, there are clues suggesting similar tick-borne illnesses have affected humans across centuries. As far back as the 19th century, conditions like "tick-borne relapsing fevers" plagued rural communities, resembling what we see with Lyme. Researchers have now retrospectively diagnosed historic cases meeting key Lyme criteria.

Indigenous traditions among communities like the Iroquois also reference stages of seasonal sickness, recounted alongside advice to avoid areas where ticks congregate during the summer months when transmission risk is highest. Without awareness of microscopic bacteria, these communities nonetheless created ecological codes and preventative measures, indicating they associated tick bites with subsequent illness.

Today, Lyme remains endemic in rural areas of the United States, Europe, and Asia—essentially anywhere ecosystems support tick and mammalian host populations. For cultures dependent on forest resources or agriculture facilitating tick habitat near human contact, warnings of tick-borne disease have echoed for centuries before medical science caught up. With climate change broadening endemic boundaries, perhaps listening to ecological wisdom about tick avoidance and signs of infection remains most relevant. Blending this with modern medicine can further evolve the dialogue around mitigating longstanding vector-borne illnesses in human history.

Common Misconceptions

Several pervasive myths about Lyme disease persist both in the medical community and in the general public, hampering efforts to direct appropriate diagnostics and treatment. These misconceptions also minimize the struggles of many Lyme patients. We must clarify the facts.

One major misconception is that Lyme testing is straightforward and highly accurate. While standard antibody screening may help confirm some acute cases, it misses 35–50% of affected patients, particularly those with later disseminated or lingering symptoms. This book will unravel the complexities and flaws of current lab diagnostics.

Another myth is that a short course of antibiotics reliably cures most Lyme. Unfortunately, the Lyme bacteria have developed clever mechanisms to evade immune attacks and resist antibiotics, often allowing it to persist despite treatment. The notion that lingering patient symptoms after treatment are merely "post-infectious" rather than due to ongoing infection is ignorant of extensive research on bacterial persistence.

Finally, attitudes framing Lyme only as an acute infection downplay the pervasive, devastating effects on patients' lives when they struggle with debilitating symptoms for years. Referring to their illness as "medically unexplained" if test results do not corroborate their experience is dismissive and compounds suffering. This book validates these lived-patient realities.

Chapter 2

The Lyme Disease Spectrum

Early-Stage Symptoms

In early localized Lyme, flu-like symptoms usually emerge within 3 to 30 days after an infected tick attaches and transmits Borrelia burgdorferi (Bb). These include fatigue, headaches, fevers, chills, muscle aches, stiff necks, and swollen lymph nodes. An expanding "bull's eye" rash at the bite location develops in about 70% of cases. If untreated, symptoms can wax and wane over the next few weeks.

As bacteria disseminate, they can affect the heart's electrical signaling, resulting in palpitations, lightheadedness, or fainting, illustrating why cardiologists need Lyme awareness. Nervous system inflammation also generates symptoms like facial palsy, numbness or tingling, and heightened pain sensitivity at this stage.

Prompt antibiotic treatment during an early infection typically resolves these symptoms for most patients. However, for reasons we will explore later, a subset of patients may experience lingering effects that form the basis of post-treatment Lyme disease syndrome. Careful clinical observation is required to determine whether additional agents or supportive interventions can help resolve persistent symptoms or if an alternate diagnosis is warranted.

Progression to Chronic Lyme

Without sufficient immune response and antibiotic treatment in the early stages, Lyme bacteria exploit stealth mechanisms, allowing them to advance infection and trigger widespread inflammatory damage, resulting in chronic Lyme disease. This systemic illness produces waxing and waning bouts of debilitating symptoms spanning inflammatory arthritis, neurological dysfunction, extreme fatigue, autonomic issues like headaches or gut irregularities, and, for some, even psychiatric manifestations.

Bb bacteria prefer connective tissue once disseminated, inhabiting joints, cardiac tissue, and even the protective myelin coating around nerves. Patients describe radiating nerve sensations or burning limbic pain as nerves come under fire. Over time, immune cells also appear to mount autoimmune reactions, worsening neurological inflammation.

Cognitive symptoms like brain fog, speech issues, and memory problems develop as infection and trauma cascade in the central nervous system. For still-unknown reasons, women make up 60–80% of chronic Lyme cases. Hormone interactions may reduce immune competence or facilitate bacterial shielding mechanisms. However the exact pathology progresses, chronic Lyme can be extremely isolating and life-limiting, necessitating comprehensive support.

Variations in Patient Experiences

While certain symptom patterns offer clues about Lyme disease progression, no two patients experience this complex illness in the same way. The disease expression can look very different depending on variables like the specific Borrelia strains involved, whether other tick-borne co-infections are also transmitted, the patient's unique genetics, lifestyle factors influencing immune function, and the stage of diagnosis or treatment.

For example, some patients may struggle predominantly with severe musculoskeletal pain and arthritis. Others contend primarily with heart arrhythmias and neuropathy. Still more grapple with neurological manifestations or destabilizing autonomic dysfunction. Many unlucky patients deal with shifting degrees of all of the above.

The duration, periodicity, and intensity of flares also vary widely. While some enjoy extended periods of remission where symptoms calm, others describe more constant battles to function through daily symptom storms. Honoring these highly personalized voices and experiences is critical as we move toward integrated care for Lyme disease. No two cases look identical, nor should treatment. We meet patients where they are while illuminating the complexity that science continues to unravel.

Chapter 3

Diagnostic Tools and Techniques

Traditional Testing Methods

Currently, the laboratory standard for diagnosing Lyme disease hinges on the serological detection of antibodies against the bacteria using an ELISA or Western Blot test. However, innate flaws with these indirect methods and problems with outdated CDC reporting criteria render them highly fallible for capturing many real Lyme cases.

Antibody tests only show a positive result after the immune system has mounted a detectable response, making early detection difficult. Because Borrelia burgdorferi bacteria are exceptionally skilled at subverting immune reactions through cloaking, cyst formation, or inhabiting immunoprotected cell niches, serum antibody presence is unpredictable, particularly in late-stage disseminated cases.

Mainstream Western Blots also utilize just one lab strain of Lyme bacteria rather than accounting for diverse strains circulating in the environment, causing cross-reactivity issues. Many specialists are now disregarding CDC surveillance criteria to clinically diagnose and treat probable Lyme disease in patients with relevant exposure histories and symptoms, which are validated by observed treatment responses. Advanced specialty labs offer more sensitive and specific testing to complement clinical findings.

Advanced Diagnostic Approaches

Given the difficulties with conventional Lyme diagnostics, integrative practitioners employ a multifaceted approach to assessing clinical presentation and specialized lab work to map the terrain of possible infection and cofactors perpetuating inflammation. They dig to understand a patient's exposures, lifestyle habits, genetic risks, and sources of physiological stress that may provide openings for illness to take root.

Important tools in the diagnostic arsenal include advanced direct microscopy searching for Borrelia structures in blood, CSF, or tissue biopsies. RNA detection through Polymerase Chain Reaction (PCR) can also help confirm an active infection. Evaluating immune markers like CD57 counts and C4a levels reveals infection-induced inflammation. Some clinicians test neurotransmitter levels or networks to assess neuropathy. Others map gut microbiome ecology.

No perfect test for every patient exists, but piecing together clinical, historical, and advanced lab insights allows functional medicine detectives to zero in on the most likely factors driving illness and perpetuating misery for a given patient. This sets the stage for comprehensive treatment of the root causes rather than just suppressing symptoms.

Challenges in Lyme Diagnosis

Pinpointing a definitive Lyme disease diagnosis can be extremely frustrating and complex for several reasons. First, the limitations of conventional antibody screening miss many cases and invite false assumptions about who warrants treatment. Patients with credible symptoms but negative ELISA or Western Blot results often get dismissed or misdiagnosed. The inaccurate notion that straightforward testing interferes with care for these neglected patients.

Secondly, Lyme has over 100 recognized symptoms that mirror many other conditions, ranging from chronic fatigue syndrome and fibromyalgia to multiple sclerosis, ALS, or various psychiatric illnesses. Patients frequently acquire multiple inaccurate diagnoses on the winding road to uncovering Lyme disease as the central culprit behind their suffering. This diagnostic confusion delays access to essential treatment.

Finally, Lyme seldom travels alone. Upwards of 40% of patients are also estimated to harbor one or more co-infecting tick-borne pathogens like Babesia, Bartonella, Mycoplasma, Anaplasma, and Rocky Mountain Spotted Fever, making causation trickier to pin down. Solving the diagnostic mystery requires recognizing patterns while accounting for complexity.

Chapter 4

Integrative Treatment Approaches

Conventional Medical Treatments

Currently, the frontline conventional approach to treating acute Lyme involves oral antibiotics like doxycycline or amoxicillin for 2-4 weeks based on severity and response, occasionally coupled with intravenously delivered drugs for disseminated cases. These regimens often resolve symptoms when deployed early after recent tick exposure and infection. However, the Lyme bacteria deploy defense tactics, allowing a surviving subset to remain behind after an antibiotic assault.

For patients with longer-term, untreated infections now manifesting chronic symptoms or those who relapse after initial antibiotic treatment and develop post-treatment Lyme disease, referred to as PTLDS or chronic Lyme, mainstream medicine often has little to offer beyond symptom management. Recommendations rarely reflect the newest science.

Lyme-literate practitioners pioneering integrative approaches use advanced diagnostics to confirm ongoing infection or inflammation and tailor-tailored treatment regimens that include pharmaceutical agents, herbal antimicrobials, nutrition, and lifestyle changes to give patients renewed hope.

Complementary and Alternative Therapies

While antibiotics have a role in attacking active Lyme infection, especially in early cases, employing them alone fails far too many suffering later-stage and chronic patients. This points to the need for multi-modal care. Lyme-literate doctors often pair pharmaceuticals like rotation antibiotics or off-label drugs alongside herbal protocols, nutrition and detox support, and lifestyle changes, providing compounded benefits.

Herbal therapies based on plants such as Japanese knotweed, cat's claw, andrographis, and garlic concentrate antimicrobial effects directly on Lyme while modulating immunity and inflammation pathways beneficial to symptom resolution. Nutrient cofactors depleted by infection, such as manganese, zinc, and magnesium, also aid recovery—detoxification aids such as glutathione precursors, saunas, lymph drainage massages, clearing bacterial debris, and neurotoxins. Gentle movement, stress relief, and sleep hygiene practices reduce flare triggers.

By assessing the dominant forces driving illness in each patient and crafting combinatorial protocols, practitioners restore function and radically improve quality of life. We now know solutions exist for many struggling Lyme patients when care centers around their lived experiences rather than outdated medical dogma or primitive, singular treatment models.

Holistic Healing Modalities

Beyond pharmaceutical and herbal interventions, incorporating holistic healing modalities as part of a comprehensive Lyme treatment plan can help calm physiological stress, reduce inflammatory drivers, and encourage immune regulation and neurological repair to pave the path for patient recovery.

Modalities like acupuncture, meditation/mindfulness practices, guided imagery/visualization, and certain movement therapies harness the power of the brain-body connection, supporting wellness. Acupuncture, in particular, has shown benefits in relieving Lyme musculoskeletal pain, neuropathy, fatigue, and brain fog by harmonizing nervous, immune, and endocrine system functioning.

Emotional or energetic approaches like spiritual counseling, Emotional Freedom Technique (EFT), or Eye Movement Desensitization and Reprocessing (EMDR) also empower patients to process trauma related to illness while stimulating profound physiological shifts. By attending to the whole patient—body, mind, and spirit—across modalities, we unlock synergistic potential for healing seemingly intractable Lyme disease.

Chapter 5

Nutritional Support for Lyme Patients

Importance of Nutrition in Lyme Treatment

While drugs and herbs play key roles in tackling active Lyme bacteria, nutrition forms an equally vital pillar powering recovery for several important reasons. First, depleted nutritional status almost always accompanies long-term infection due to impaired absorption, inflammatory damage, and medication side effects, undermining healing.

Next, nutrients like Vitamins C and D, which most Lyme patients lack, have direct anti-microbial effects and immune-regulatory activities that optimize bacterial clearance. Minerals, including zinc, manganese, and molybdenum, act as essential cofactors, driving hundreds of detoxification and antioxidant enzymes required to mitigate infection-induced inflammation and neurotoxin damage that maintain symptoms.

Prebiotic and probiotic foods to repair the gut microbiome also grow more relevant as researchers uncover links between gut permeability ("leaky gut"), heightened inflammation, and bacterial translocation risks across that barrier—all prevalent in Lyme. Pursuing a brain- and gut-nourishing anti-inflammatory diet low in immune-reactive foods accelerates progress.

Nutritional biochemistry is the foundation for determining how effectively the body marshals its healing forces. An integrated care plan succeeds or fails on the power of this foundation.

Dietary Guidelines

Optimizing nutrition for Lyme disease entails emphasizing whole, anti-inflammatory foods while minimizing intake of pro-inflammatory agricultural products and processed items. Key guidelines include:

- Focus on certified organic fruits, vegetables, herbs, and spices; ethically raised meats; and sustainable seafood to maximize nutrient content and avoid pesticide exposures that stress detox pathways. Eat the rainbow, seeking variety. Choose low-glycemic index options to stabilize blood sugar.
- Embrace healthy fats like olive oil, avocado, nuts and seeds, and omega-3-rich seafood, which promote cell membrane integrity and hormone balance. Avoid refined vegetable or seed oils.
- Minimize sugar, excess starchy grains, conventional dairy, factory-farmed meat, and artificial additives that spur inflammation. Most should eliminate gluten.
- Stay well hydrated with filtered water, herbal tea, and bone broth; the right fluids flush toxins and support every healing process in the body.
- Listen to your body and adjust serving sizes and proportions to fit your current state and health goals. Mindful, soothing practices while eating also encourage proper digestion and assimilation.

Through dietary tweaks reducing inflammatory drivers and boosting micronutrients, the groundwork transforms to help anti-microbial and detox efforts progress Lyme treatment.

Supplements and Nutraceuticals

While whole foods should form the foundation of nutritional plans for Lyme patients, targeted supplementation with essential vitamins, minerals, antioxidants, and plant-derived compounds often provides additional benefits supporting healing processes. Key categories to consider include:

1. **Anti-microbial:** herbs like Andrographis, cat's claw, resveratrol, berberine, and monolaurin
2. **Anti-inflammatory:** Curcumin, MSM, fish oil, quercetin, magnesium, and NAC
3. **Antioxidants:** Vitamin C, glutathione precursors, alpha-lipoic acid
4. **Micronutrients:** B vitamins, zinc, manganese, vitamin D, and CoQ10.
5. **GI Support:** Probiotics, marshmallows, licorice, slippery elm
6. **Neuroprotectants:** Ginkgo, acetyl l-carnitine, glycine, and theanine

Dosage should be adjusted based on laboratory testing that identifies areas of deficiency, oxidative stress and inflammation levels, and microbiome status that may benefit from targeted nutraceutical combinations designed by integrative specialists. Nutrition or nutrition-based medical care providers.

Chapter 6

Mind-Body Connection in Lyme Healing

Psychosocial Impact of Lyme Disease

As a complex, systemic condition with tentacles pervading nearly every bodily system and domain of health, living with Lyme and its episodic flares over months or years often exerts massive emotional, cognitive, and psychosocial tolls that are most underestimated unless personally experiencing this illness marathon.

Between battling often debilitating physical symptoms affecting stamina, wresting with brain fog, word-finding troubles, and short-term memory gaps that hamper

|| 29 ||

communication, struggling to fulfill roles, responsibilities, and dreams forfeited to illness, and lacking validation about the seriousness and physiological basis of symptoms from uninformed medical providers and social contacts, the predicament strains mental health and tests the inner compass guiding resilience.

Anger, grief, isolation, depression, and anxiety frequently emerge. Self-concept crumbles for those who were previously high performers. Trust in health systems fractures. Financial standing may pivot. Relationships come under fire or are lifelines if nurtured with care and empathy. Learning to navigate this psychological and social terrain proves vital but is underemphasized.

Mindfulness and Stress Reduction

Finding ways to cultivate mindfulness and consciously work to shift mindset and manage stressful triggers proves pivotal in managing Lyme and preventing symptom flares that otherwise readily emerge in fight-or-flight states when the nervous system is on overdrive.

Techniques like meditation, deep breathing, guided visualization, being present in nature, prayer, writing in a journal, sensory grounding practices, enjoyable hobbies, and setting healthy boundaries and expectations for what your current body state can handle all build resilience. Some benefit from support groups sharing wisdom. Light yoga, tai chi, qigong, and other gentle movement modalities also train mindfulness through bodily awareness.

The mindset piece involves learning radical self-acceptance and self-compassion—coming to terms with grief for lives derailed by illness while actively reframing stories we tell about controllability. Rather than battling the body, we must learn to be non-judgmentally attuned to its cues and craft a lifestyle in alignment. Psychotherapy helps some unpack trauma and develop helpful mental habits.

Integrating Mental Health into Treatment

Far too often, psychological aspects of navigating chronic Lyme disease are glanced over or extracted from biomedical treatment plans despite extensive research confirming mind-body interactions shape illness trajectories through mechanisms like the gut-brain axis, HPA stress responses, neurotransmitter tone, and nerve signaling modulation via neuropeptides and electrical frequencies.

As such, practitioners committed to holistic Lyme treatment must learn to ask questions illuminating contributing mental health factors and include therapies directly targeting stress physiology, pharmaceuticals, and nutrition approaches in their integrated care models. Tracking relevant metrics like heart rate variability, inflammatory markers, sleep quality, and questionnaires about anxiety and depression should accompany standard lab orders to capture patient experiences.

Some patients benefit from psychological counseling or techniques like EMDR and biofeedback that retrain nervous system responses. Community-based support groups offer the connections that are missing when one is solitary due to illness. There is no healing in isolation. Recognizing areas where additional behavioral health support may accelerate Lyme recoveries will elevate patient outcomes and quality of life. Healing the whole patient demands no less.

Chapter 7

Prevention Strategies

Tick Avoidance and Safety Measures

Preventing tickborne illness begins with strategic tick avoidance, especially when venturing outdoors in wooded, bushy, or grassy habitats where vector numbers concentrate between April and September. Key measures include:

- Wear light-colored clothing, enabling you to spot ticks easily.
- Tuck pants into socks when walking through high brush or grass.
- Consider treating clothing or shoes designed to repel or kill ticks.

- Use EPA-registered DEET or natural repellents on exposed skin.
- Stay in the center of trails when hiking, avoiding brushing vegetation.

Create tick-safe zones in your yard through woodchip barriers, trimming vegetation, and deterrent plantings.

When returning indoors, conduct tick checks and safely remove any found using fine-tipped tweezers grasping close to mouth parts near the skin without squeezing the body. Disinfect the bite site afterward and monitor for signs of rash over the next several days. Catching ticks quickly prevents transmission in most cases.

Immunization Research and Development

While no human Lyme disease vaccine currently exists after earlier attempts failed and were pulled from the market, promising research continues exploring new candidate formulations aiming to trigger a protective antibody response against common Borrelia antigens before an infection occurs.

One vaccine candidate, VLA15, focusing on outer surface protein A, is now in phase 3 of human trials, showing strong immunogenicity and helping clear bacteria in animal models. Researchers are also examining the potential for Bilderback's mysterious LYMErix vaccine to cause adverse autoimmune reactions in some people. Significantly advancing detection capabilities and unlocking biomarkers of protection will help next-generation vaccines skirt past pitfalls.

Innovations enabling accurate differentiation between prior environmental exposure and current active infection also need refining so vaccination does not complicate diagnosis through false positives. Safely evoking durable, reliable immunity against diverse Borrelia strains with one vaccination remains the holy grail. However, with revived biopharma interest, cautious optimism exists that breakthrough preventions are on the horizon before the end of the decade.

Community Education and Advocacy

With Lyme disease diagnoses escalating and sizable gaps persisting around public familiarity with risks, prevention, and pathways to accessing accurate diagnosis and treatment, grassroots community education and advocacy efforts remain instrumental in influencing trajectories at local, state, and national levels.

Patient-led organizations, such as the Lyme Disease Association, work tirelessly to expand educational offerings for schools and community groups while advocating for healthcare policy and research funding reforms that are critical to driving progress. Local in-person support groups allow newly diagnosed patients to be mentored to navigate complex terrain.

Passionate advocacy organizations give voice to struggles that would otherwise go unheard and drive transformations that catalyze a healthier future for all at risk of tick-borne diseases through online information sharing, in-person demonstrations, and relationship building, spurring endorsed legislation protecting patient access to integrative care options while opposing rigid institutions unwilling to update flawed protocols.

Chapter 8

Looking Toward the Future

Emerging Research and Innovations

As Lyme disease diagnosis and debilitating patient experiences continue to rise despite standard treatments, research momentum, and biotech innovations are finally gaining steam to deliver next-generation solutions serving unmet needs.

In addition to new vaccines, increased NIH funding has resulted in many advances in detection methods, such as direct microscopy techniques, metabolomics biomarkers that will allow early diagnosis before antibodies appear, and rapid nanotechnology platforms that can detect infection with just one drop of blood within minutes, which is a significant advancement over current antibody-based assays.

Expanded clinical trials are also investigating existing pharmaceutical agents like disulfiram, which show promise for clearing persistent bacteria when conventional regimens fail. New insights around dysregulated immune networks and infection-induced autoimmunity also inform the pipeline of immunomodulatory drugs that may soon help refractory patients.

While no magic bullet exists to address every patient scenario given Lyme's complexities, the burgeoning knowledge gains and technology-assisted detection and treatment developments underway provide real hope that therapeutic futures will burn brighter for thousands locked in struggles today.

The Role of Technology in Lyme Management

Consumer-facing and point-of-care technologies stand to transform early Lyme detection, disease tracking, treatment support, and patient experiences navigating a formidable illness.

In the diagnosis realm, next-generation wearable insect tracking devices will geo-tag locations, warning individuals about tick exposure risks and prompting preventative measures before bites occur. At-home test kits and smartphone-synced diagnostics will accelerate early lab confirmation, moving monitoring out of hospitals and into homes.

Digital apps that track symptoms are already helping patients keep track of flare-ups and new patterns so that they can be analyzed in the future. Machine learning systems help connect factors that make symptoms worse or better, which allows for group decisions. Such data will feed large-scale disease registries, spotlighting where research and clinical gaps exist through real-world evidence.

As telemedicine infrastructure expands post-pandemic, underserved patient populations may also gain access to distant specialty providers through virtual conduits, connecting those with the right expertise to guide individualized care plans otherwise locally lacking.

Building a Lyme-Resilient Future

Lyme and associated tickborne diseases are fast becoming ubiquitous threads in the fabric of modern life for individuals living, working, and playing across habitats prime for transmitting Borrelia. Our greatest hope rests in galvanizing coordinated large-scale momentum around research, innovation, policy reforms, environmental stewardship, and grassroots education essential to bend the curve and rewrite risky trajectories.

More government and private research funding is needed to support the development of diagnostics, new treatments, training programs for specialized care providers, health equity initiatives, and investments in figuring out what we still do not know about how vectors behave and how their environments change as the climate changes.

Updating screening guidelines and medical education priorities to encourage more accurate and timely diagnoses, along with insurance reforms that make integrative care options more available, would also help avoid nightmare scenarios in which more and more patients suffer from painful symptoms that will not go away. Prevention through emerging immunization options and tick control methods in public spaces must be addressed, too.

Ultimately, by elevating awareness, empowering individuals, supporting healers and innovators, and interweaving medical, environmental, and community-centered breakthroughs, we manifest the conditions that make Lyme disease management a surmountable challenge rather than a basis for despair. The ingredients for change are within reach through a unified vision and values prioritizing compassion.

Conclusion

One clear conclusion follows from examining the intricacies of Lyme disease mysteries and the reasons for growing optimism in the field of research: outdoor enthusiasts, patients, doctors, caregivers, and advocates must collaborate to demand and support important innovations that replace outmoded paradigms that do not meet needs, as demonstrated by the alarmingly high rates of post-treatment chronic suffering and the soaring diagnosis rates.

For far too long, institutional gatekeeping has prevented rigid stances from being updated, and those still battling opt-debilitating constellations of symptoms exist primarily in their minds rather than the persistence of matrix-entrenched spirochetes resistant to brief antimicrobial monotherapy.

These approaches not only alienate patients; they prevent researchers from recognizing tenable contributors perpetuating widespread misery and navigation hurdles delaying access to life-changing interventions until late-stage disruption takes a grip, forcing disability or early retirement.

However, modern scientific insights around vector behaviors in a climate-shifting world, microscopy techniques piercing cloaking tactics, genomic signaling pathways disrupted, enabling immune system sabotage, and cellular locales bunkered safely out of antibiotic reach. Pharmaceutical, herbal, and nutraceutical compound synergies have now shed light on the possibility of lingering pathogen reservoirs or secondary conditions caused by acute-stage infection.

Emerging diagnostic technologies go beyond dated antibody-based assays and bidirectional brain pilot mishaps; immunome tabulations catalog precise glitches caused by antigen trickery; and pharmacological cream-of-the-crop trials employ unique disruption abilities, selectively severing lifeline nutrients from stealth microbes while avoiding typical front-line antibiotic gauntlets.

However, mapping the territory where physiology, ecology, and microbiology intersect remains simply the starting point. Genuine change requires that medical institutions foster environments in which empathetic, multidisciplinary practitioners have leeway in codesigning therapeutic journeys that account for patients' lived expertise rather than dismissiveness of contested complaints lacking straightforward confirmatory lab evidence.

It requires flexible insurance systems to adequately compensate clinicians, carving space for practicing integrative investigative medicine, and amalgamating benefits from conventional and functional lenses.

Creating regional centers for specialized care, developing skills in navigating complex webs of symptoms shared by communities, stewardship of grassroots resources such as peer mentoring programs, school educational pilots, municipal land management policies limiting rodent reservoirs in public recreation areas, and reforming pop culture by eliminating antiquated tropes and making jokes about "chronic Lyme" will not result in societal progress.

In essence, creating a Lyme-resilient world demands commitment, fostering health literacy, and catalyzing innovation and cooperation from bedside to bench to backyard. Though no quick fixes or guaranteed cures may exist, this book illuminates Bacon's guiding direction if social action will activate around the cause. Perhaps most critically, it gives voice to validating struggles that otherwise individual, marginalized, and medicalized spawn further isolation. You deserve radically better. We all do.

Only together, by naming collective responsibility while mining and integrating our finest human attributes of compassion, critical thinking, and ingenuity, may we rupture assumptions, consigning populations to gray zones of misery falling through fragmented systemic cracks, ultimately serving each other and future generations through wisdom hard-earned on the crucible and walking this path first.

www.ingramcontent.com/pod-product-compliance
Lightning Source LLC
Chambersburg PA
CBHW062303290526
45794CB00006B/2681